WATER DETOX AND INTERMITTENT FASTING

FOR: GENERAL BODY HEALTH, WEIGTH LOSS, INFLAMMATORY DISEASES, HIGH BLOOD PRESSURE, AGING, CANCER PREVENTION

Dr Scott Tyler

DEDICATION

This work is dedicated to the Almighty God who is the source of good health.

CONTENTS

ACKNOWLEDGMENTS

This is to acknowledge the pains and worries of all those suffering from chronic illnesses. Please be rest assured that you are not alone in your struggles, as I pray God to stretch His healing hand upon you.

PART ONE

GENERAL INTRODUCTION

Life can be long, healthy and wonderful. This is possible in part when we make the right choices. These choices are invariably results of our thoughts and emotions. If we make good choices, we would reap the fruits at harvest time which can be in the short or long term. These choices we make very soon form the body of habits we have. There is no gainsaying then that it is imperative to force upon ourselves habits are good, wholesome and positive.

It is timely to remember that a tree is known and judged by its fruits. The single most important habit we must form to succeed in life is without a doubt, self discipline. Self discipline can be targeted at personal life, business, religion or whatever goal(s) that we set out to achieve. The ways by which we intend to practice this discipline vary as the goal varies. Some goals require that we travel by more than one way.

For instance, for someone who has the goal of success in business, these questions pop up: what will the ideal business look like? What needs would you be aiming to satisfy? What sort of set up would you create? What position would you occupy? How much would be your turnover in a week, month, and year? What caliber of people would you employ and deal with? And what would you really need to do begin doing or refrain from doing to achieve this set ideal? Such a person might need to practice habits such as self discipline as regards studying books and materials that business people require, investing and attending relevant training sessions intended for business oriented people, avail oneself for possible meetings with top business executives, practice patterns of thinking like business people do. For such a person, the ways are multiple. And only faithfulness in most of all of these ways would count.

For someone whose goal is good health, these questions would be the burden: what will this health state look like? What should be the optimal weight? What would differentiate the ideal health you seek from the health you enjoy or suffer presently? What pertinent measures or habits need to be developed to help you achieve the ideal health? The ways or habits you need to develop might include studying about health, refraining from rough activity such as fighting, keeping tabs on excesses of food and drink, fasting, etc. Here again we see that the ways or the habits are multiple. The necessity of forming habits is simply one thing we cannot escape no matter how hard we try. It is so natural that the failure to form habits that are good and profiting is itself habit in one form or another.

All good habits are hard to form, no doubt, but they are easy to live with, so says Brain Tracy. Within this book we have dealt exhaustively with the habit of fasting.

PART TWO: FASTING AND ITS HEALTH BENEFITS

2.1   INTRODUCTION

In this first part of this book, we shall be dealing broadly with the concept of fasting. Fasting is basically a form of abstinence for some goal. This is in keeping with the assertion by Aristotle that every action is thought to aim at some goal which can be happiness, profit, well being, the good or pleasure. Apart from this, there are a couple of reasons that push our need to fast which include religion, good health, etc.

There are myths that have been posited around fasting. Many of these myths are exaggerations of the truth as others are plain cases of falsehood. Well, a myth is always a myth and there will always be myths so long as humans are involved. Finally in this part, we shall introduce five types of fast which we shall develop in later parts. We shall introduce religious, intermittent, juice/calorie restriction, partial and water fasts.

We shall look at the gains of fasting with particular emphasis to gains such as insulin resistance reduction, victory over inflammation, improvement of blood pressure, boost of brain function, limitation of calorie intake, enhancement of growth hormone secretion, delayed aging, and cancer prevention. Thereafter we shall discuss the side effects of fasting in general.

2.2   WHAT IS FASTING?

Fasting is widely considered as the conscious abstinence or reduction from all or some of food, drink, or both, for a specified period of time. An absolute fast (dry fasting) is normally defined as abstinence from all food and liquid for a definite period. Other kinds of fasts may be in some measure restrictive, cutting down on only particular foods or substances, or be intermittent.

When looked at physiologically, fasting can also refer to the metabolic status of a person who has not eaten through the night, or to the metabolic state achieved after full digestion and absorption of a meal. Several metabolic adjustments occur during fasting. It is possible to use diagnostic tests to measure any state of fasting. Some diagnostic tests are used to determine a fasting state. For example, a person is generally assumed to be fasting once 8–12 hours have gone by since the last meal. Metabolic change of the fasting state is considered to have begun after absorption of a meal (typically 3–5 hours after eating).

Diagnostic fasts are fasts that extended till about 70 hours but it is important to ensure that strict care is put into properly investigate any health complications. Many people may also fast as a requirement for a medical procedure, such as preceding a colonoscopy or a checkup. Fasting, more broadly, may also be part of a religious ritual. This religious aspect is actually the driving force behind the sustenance of the concept and practice of fasting.

For those who are booked for surgery or other medical procedures, fasting is recommended because they require general anesthesia because of the threat of pulmonary aspiration of gastric contents after induction of anesthesia (i.e., vomiting and inhaling the vomit, causing life-threatening aspiration pneumonia). Furthermore, certain medical tests, such as cholesterol testing (lipid panel) or certain blood glucose measurements necessitate fasting for several hours so that a baseline can be established. In the case of a lipid panel, refusal to fast for a full 12 hours (including vitamins) will guarantee an elevated triglyceride measurement.

Fasting often improves mood, alertness, and personal feelings of well-being, perhaps improving overall symptoms of depression. Fasting for durations shorter than 24 hours (intermittent fasting) has been shown to be effectual for weight loss in obese and healthy adults and to preserve lean body mass.

It has widely believed that fasting makes one more appreciative of food. In chance occurrences, fasting can lead to re-feeding syndrome.

Fasting when one peers into history has often been employed as a tool to protest, make a political statement, or to bring awareness to a cause. A hunger strike, a non-violent method of resistance, is often staged as an act of political protest, or to rouse feelings of guilt, or to attain a goal such as a policy change. A spiritual fast presupposes personal spiritual beliefs with the need to express personal principles, from time to time in the context of a social injustice.

Mohandas K. Gandhi, the political and religious leader, undertook several long fasts as political and social protests. His fasts had a noteworthy impact on the British Raj and the Indian population generally.

Bobby Sands was a prisoner in Northern Ireland; he was part of the 1981 Irish hunger strike that was aimed at bringing about better rights in prison. Sands had just won election to the British Parliament but rather tragically died after 66 days of complete fast. Remarkably, his funeral was attended by 100,000 people and the ongoing strike only came to its terminus after nine other men died. In all, ten brave and determined men survived without food for 46 to 73 days.

César Chávez carried out numerous spiritual fasts, including a 25-day fast in 1968 advancing the principle of nonviolence, and a fast christened 'thanksgiving and hope' in preparation for pre-set civil disobedience by farm workers. Chávez strongly considered a spiritual fast as a spiritual transformation that was highly personal. Other forward looking campaigns have adopted the scheme.

2.3   WHY FAST?

The human race has in reality been fasting for a very good number of years. Often times it was carried out of necessity, once there simply was not any food available. In some cases, it was made for religious reasons. A good number of religions, Islam, Christianity and Buddhism inclusive, authorize some form of fasting.

The human race and other animals inclusive tend to often impulsively fast when sick. Undoubtedly, there is not anything unnatural about fasting, and our bodies are very well equipped biologically to cope with the harsh reality of prolonged periods of not eating. All kinds of processes in the body are modified on the occasion that we don't eat for a while, so as to give room for our bodies to thrive during a regime of famine. It has to do with genes, hormones and important cellular repair processes. After a fast, we register considerable reductions in blood sugar and insulin levels, as well as a radical increase in human growth hormone.

There are many people carry out intermittent fasting solely to lose weight, as it is a very simple and effectual way to curb calories and burn fat. Many others indulge in it for the metabolic health gains, as it can perk up various diverse risk factors and health indicators. Pointedly, there is also a number of evidence that buttress the fact that intermittent fasting can aid you live longer. Studies carried out in rodents reveal that it can lengthen lifespan as effectively as calorie restriction. Still some research also put forward that it can facilitate protection against diseases, including Alzheimer's disease, heart disease, cancer, type 2 diabetes, and others. Other groups basically like the expediency of intermittent fasting.

It is a valuable personal practice which makes your life simpler, while augmenting your health simultaneously. The fewer meals you need to plan for, the simpler your life will be. Not having to eat for three to four times per day, taking into consideration the usual amount of preparation that goes just for cooking and cleaning that comes afterwards, also saves time. A lot of it. Humans are well tailored to fasting from time to time. Modern research shows that it has benefits for weight loss, metabolic health, and disease prevention and may even help you live longer.

2.4 FASTING MYTHS

Before any exposition is done it is not out of place to first consider the general perception of people concerning this matter. This also will help situate the mind of the reader as to reason why fasting isn't as crazy as you think it is. There are a lot of people getting things wrong because of prevailing subjective or uneducated claims. That being said, if you're already happy with your health and do not see much room for improvement, then feel free to still consider some of what will follow because there are a lot of myths surrounding the concept and practice of fasting. First some or all of the following myths to be considered will hold water if fasting was mandatory for everyone. We make bold to affirm that it is not something mandatory for anyone; rather it is just another method among the general methodologies of life that can be handy for some people. Broadly, there are beliefs that fasting may not be as valuable for the female folk as men, and it may reveal itself as an unfortunate alternative for people who are easily acclimatized to eating disorders. First read how we address each of these myths and then you can you decide if to try this out. No matter the clarification and justification we give for fasting, there is no gainsaying that calories still count, and food quality is still absolutely crucial.

First myth, fasting is simply some new fad or crazy marketing ploy. Fasting has been practiced by various religious groups for centuries. Professionals in the fields of medicine, psychology and religion among others have repeatedly affirmed the health benefits of fasting for thousands of years now. In other words, the efficacy of fating as a practice that holds many mental, physical and spiritual gains has been proven by widespread usage and the passage of time. It has been around for a long time and it is actually efficacious.

Second myth, fasting is quite foreign to many on the reason that is has never been a trendy topic. You must realize the most profound of things are hardly trendy topics. The actuating force behind this is simply the fact that nobody stands to smile to bank by telling you to not purchase what they sell, consume what they produce or even try out the supplements they market. Hence, fasting is not a very marketable topic. This explains on another level why it is not trendy especially for advertising and marketing. This leaves fasting as an obscure and arcane practice, even though it really is not.

Third myth, your body is meant to be nourished always. Inadvertently, we all have fasted in one way or another, for one simple reason or out of compulsion; you may just have not realized so. For instance, you have slept late on Saturday and ended up having your first meal of the day on Sunday after noon because you were in church. For some people, this is the practice every weekend. Have you had to travel or work and as a result did not get the time to splurge on a meal only to end up missing two to three meals consecutively? This is common for most people. In such circumstances, you had an 8hour, 16 hour or even a 24 hour fast but you did not realize.

Final myth, when you miss a meal you body is cheated and it will surely bring harm to you. It is true that we need to eat to survive. This does not mean that we live to eat, we only eat to live. There are instances of certain fasting in daily life to counteract this myth. The health benefits that come with fasting would not have been possible if we were meant to keeping living only if we ate.

2.5   FASTING TYPES

There are many different types of fasts, so the exercise of finding a worthy method that fits your lifestyle is made easier with increasing options. This same advantage can be put many at the crossroads anyway.

Here are a few of the most common types of fasting which we shall discuss in details in a short while:

- **Water   fasting:** Necessitates consuming just water within a period specifically set aside for this. It can vary from a few hours to a couple of days.
- **Religious fasting**: requires that you fast for   reasons   of   religion.   Spiritual demands often bring up instances that mandate that we fast for a short while in a day or for many couple of days.

- **Intermittent fasting:** compels that ingestion from top to bottom is regulated for fixed periods of time at a time and a typical diet is picked up again on other days.

- **Calorie restriction:** requires that calorie intake is controlled for a set number of days each week. This can even take the form of a juice fast. A juice fast is simple but requires some planning to ensure you get enough vitamins and minerals from a variety of fresh fruits and vegetables. A blend of fruit or vegetables is mixed with water and consumed three to six times daily.

- **Partial fasting:** involves the total removal of definite natural foods or processed foods, this includes drinks, animal products such as egg, milk and meat from the diet for a set period.

Enclosed within these broad groups of fasting are also more specific types of fasts. For a case in point, it is possible to break down intermittent fasting into subgroups, for instance alternate-day fasting or time-restricted feeding, involving food intake every other day and giving rise to restriction in eating to just a few hours each day respectively.

From the foregoing it has been demonstrated that there subsists bountiful ways to put into practice fasting, which makes possible a sure easy prospect to unearth a practice that is appropriate for just about any way of life. What is expected is that you try out sundry types to arrive upon what works excellently for you. For seasoned fasters, breaking down their fasting regimen into specific sub types and varying them accordingly does not present any challenge. For starters, the case is different; hence it is prudent to try experimenting with dissimilar types of fasting in a bid to settle upon what method or combination of methods best suits.

Fasting, which is practiced for an assortment of reasons, includes but is not restricted to cleansing, detoxification, weight loss, treatment of a medical condition and conformation to religious practices. As pointed out before now the type of fast you settle upon should be appropriate for your level of health, age, body make up and any special physical challenges you may have. Prior to starting a fast, discuss with your doctor or health care provider, particularly if you are on any drug regime or have a severe health state.

2.6   THE GENERAL GAINS

The Pentecostals have invariably encouraged the recent surge in popularity of the efficacy of fasting, this notwithstanding the fact that fasting as a practice dates back centuries and from our submissions on the concept of fasting above it is abundantly clear that fasting plays a central role in many cultures and religions. From the abundant positions different cultures and religions have held on fasting, one can glean basically that fasting is the abstinence from all or some foods or drinks for a set period of time. Now as there are many different traditions of fasting, there are many different ways of fasting. We shall carefully expatiate on the different types later on. In general, most types of fasts are performed over 24–72 hours. How beneficial is fasting? Can fasting reap fruits that are worth the abstinence? Fasting has been demonstrated to have many benefits particularly health benefits, these health benefits range from increased weight loss to better brain function.

1. Reduces Insulin Resistance
Several researches have established that fasting may improve blood sugar control, which could be especially handy for those on the

verge of diabetes. It is often agreed that among people with type 2 diabetes, short-term intermittent fasting significantly decreased their blood sugar levels. Although, other views posit that that both intermittent fasting and alternate-day fasting were as effective as limiting calorie intake at reducing insulin resistance. So many persons do not realize that decreasing insulin resistance can amplify your body's sensitivity to insulin; this eventually allows it to convey glucose from your bloodstream to your cells more efficiently. With the already stressed potential blood sugar-lowering effects of fasting, it can also help keep your blood sugar steady, preventing spikes and crashes in your blood sugar levels. It is important not to forget that there are studies which have found that fasting may impact blood sugar levels differently for men and women. Two type of fasting can help remedy this situation. Intermittent fasting and alternate-day fasting could help decrease blood sugar levels and reduce insulin resistance but may affect men and women differently.

2. Fights Inflammation
At the same time as acute inflammation is a normal immune process the human body uses to help fight off infections, chronic

inflammation is known to have serious consequences for your health. Several researches show that inflammation may be involved in the development of chronic conditions, such as cancer. Different efforts have demonstrated that fasting can help diminish levels of inflammation and help encourage better health. It is equally factual that observing healthy adults showed that intermittent fasting for one month appreciably decreased levels of inflammatory markers. This is correlated by another study that discovered the same end product when people fasted for 12 hours a day for one month. In addition to this, one animal study found that adhering to a very low-calorie diet to imitate the consequence of fasting reduced levels of inflammation and was beneficial in the treatment of a chronic inflammatory condition. It has equally true that fasting could lessen several markers of inflammation and may be useful in treating inflammatory conditions.

3. Improves Blood Pressure

Heart disease is well thought-out as leading basis of death around the world, the toll from this account has been estimated at 33.4% of deaths globally. Remodeling your diet and lifestyle is key and can be regarded as one of the most effectual ways to reduce your risk of heart disease. Some factual revelations from some research have strongly suggested that incorporating fasting into your routine may be especially beneficial when it comes to heart health. It is indicative that faithfulness to a regimen of eight week alternate day fast can help reduce disturbingly high levels of "unhealthy" LDL cholesterol and blood triglycerides remarkably. In a separate study whose study population consisted 110 obese adults showed that fasting for three weeks under medical supervision significantly decreased blood pressure, as well as levels of blood triglycerides. With a decrease in the foregoing, total cholesterol and "unhealthy" LDL cholesterol also reduces. In addition, people largely associated fasting with a lower risk of coronary artery disease, together with a significantly lower the danger of diabetes, which is a major threat factor for heart disease. In brief, fasting has been linked with a lower risk of coronary heart disease and may facilitate more instances of triglycerides, lower blood pressure, and cholesterol levels.

4. Boost Brain Function

Several studies have found that fasting could have a powerful effect on brain health, the only drawback here been that much of this research has been on animals and that in itself is promising but nonetheless limiting. For instance, one of such studies carried out on mice revealed that practicing intermittent fasting for over 10 months improved both brain function and brain structure. It is not only this effect of brain function improvement alone that fasting achieves, other animal studies have reported that fasting could guard brain health and augment the generation of nerve cells to help boost cognitive function. It has been established that fasting could also lend a hand in relieving inflammation, it may also support in preventing disorders that are of the neurodegenerative class. More pointedly, studies have suggested that fasting may protect against and improve outcomes for conditions such as Alzheimer's disease and Parkinson's. However, there is no gainsaying that more detailed studies are required to weigh up the effects of fasting on brain function in humans. But at the moment, research has been limited to animal studies show that fasting could improve brain function, increase nerve cell synthesis and protect against neurodegenerative conditions, such as Alzheimer's disease and Parkinson's.

5. Limits Calorie Intake

Fasting has the capacity to increase metabolism. This in turn aid safeguard muscle tissue to lessen body weight and body fat. In the same vein, it has been discovered that short-term fasting does boost metabolism by increasing amounts of the neurotransmitter norepinephrine, these often fasten up weight loss. A number of dieters turn to fasting since they are in search for a short cut that is both a fast and easy medium to drop a few pounds. Essentially, refraining from certain food classes and especially beverages ought to reduce your levels of overall calorie intake, this cascades into subsequent increased weight loss ultimately. Factually, one study revealed that whole-day fasting has capacity to reduce body weight by up to 10% thereby remarkably causing a reduction in body fat over 12–24 weeks. Penultimately, a review established that intermittent fasting for a couple of weeks was as successful in stirring up weight loss in the same vein that continuous calorie restriction and decreased body weight by about 10% and fat mass by up to 20%. In essence, fasting has been found to be more effective than calorie restriction at increasing fat loss while simultaneously preserving muscle tissue.

6. Enhance Growth Hormone Secretion

Research reveals that fasting can amplify levels of human growth hormone, a significant protein hormone that plays a vital part in growth, muscle strength, metabolism, and weight loss. Human growth hormone is a type of protein hormone that is essential to many aspects of your health. In fact, it has been established that this key hormone is involved in weight loss, growth, muscle strength, and metabolism. Many a review has demonstrated that fasting can naturally boost human growth hormone levels. In healthy adults whose diets are low in calorie, fasting for 24 hours extensively increases levels of human growth hormone. A small study consisting selected men showed that fasting for just over forty eight hours nonstop led to a 5-fold boost in the human growth hormone production rate. In addition, fasting has the capacity to ensure steady blood sugar and insulin levels throughout the hours of such fast. It is this occurrence that further optimizes levels of human growth hormone; this is consistent with reviews that have found that maintaining increased levels of insulin may lessen human growth hormone levels.

7. Delays Aging

In animals, there have been irrefutable proofs of the promise laden results on the potential lifespan-extending properties of fasting. In one specific review, rats that were subjected to fasting of the alternate day pattern experienced a delayed rate of aging and generally lived about 85% more than those who were subjected to same fasting regimens. The proposition that fasting delays ageing has been corroborated by several other studies, they conclude that fasting could be effective in increasing longevity and survival levels. Nevertheless, it is important to stress here that up to date research is still restricted to animal studies. Human related studies are considered necessary to understand how fasting may impact longevity and aging in humans. Animal studies have established that fasting may well impede aging and add to longevity, but as observed, human related research is still deficient.

8. Aids Cancer Prevention

Man is faced with the disturbing wave of cancer. As there are cells in the human body so can there be cancer as cancer simply put is abnormal cell growth. Studies on animals indicate that fasting may benefit the treatment and prevention of cancer. In fact, one of such study found that alternate-day fasting helped arrest tumor formation. Similarly, in one of the studies talked about above, it is established that exposing cancer cells to more than a few cycles of fasting was as effectual as chemotherapy in slowing down tumor growth and making the effectiveness greater than before of chemotherapy drugs on cancer development. Regrettably, nearly every one of current literature and research is narrowed to the effects of fasting on cancer formation in animals and cells. Notwithstanding these findings of great potential, supplementary studies are desirable to be looked at how fasting could sway cancer expansion and treatment in humans. In summary, some animal and test-tube studies put it to researchers that fasting could obstruct tumor development and increase the efficiency of chemotherapy.

2.7 FASTING AND ITS SIDE EFFECTS

Fasting is a procedure that has been connected with a wide variety of latent health benefits, including weight loss, as well as enhanced brain function, heart health, improved blood sugar control and cancer prevention. There are many different types of fasting that are suitable for nearly every lifestyle, from water fasting to intermittent fasting and calorie restriction. When appended with a nutritious diet and fit lifestyle, integrating fasting into your schedule could greatly benefit your health.

There is an important caveat to be conscious about at all times. Countless research and real life experiences have repeatedly demonstrated and attested to the efficacy of fasting and while it possible to make long list of would-be health reward related to fasting, nevertheless it may not be appropriate for every person. Fasting can pilot occasions of quick rises and unexpected drops in your blood sugar rates, this is particularly true of persons who are plagued by diabetes or low blood sugar, which could be precarious. It is worthwhile to first consult with your doctor if you have any not so noticeable health conditions or are planning to fast for more than 24 hours. In addition, fasting is not basically advocated particularly for older adults except accompanied by medical regulation, this extends to adolescents or people who are underweight. When such groups of people decide to try fasting, it is mandatory that they be sure to remain well-hydrated and pack their diet with nutrient-dense foods during their eating periods to take full advantage of the potential health profits.

Additionally, it is advised to, if fasting for prolong periods, try to decrease all extreme physical activity and make sure to get sufficient rest.

PART THREE: WATER FASTING

3.1   INTRODCTION

Fasting is nothing new. As we showed in the proceeding part, is has a long history particularly within religious lines. Many religious communities for centuries have had fasting as a sine qua non in their daily lives. There have been fasting diets and these were quite popular. Long before fasting became popular for health or fitness reasons, fasting was (and still is) practiced for religious or spiritual reasons.

People and companies who promote fasting often use the religious example as an explanation as to why extended fasting is healthy and acceptable. In this present day, there are countless offers to attract someone to try detoxing diets with claims of helping you achieve better health, thorough body cleansing and even the promotion of weight loss. Their selling point is often the accounts of others who have tried these diets. Some critics claim that there are no studies to back this only word of mouth.

The foregoing criticism notwithstanding, there are quite a number of clear benefits that water fasting can and does bring to the table. For water fasting, science and countless studies have demonstrated this. The only drawback has been the limitation of such studies to largely animals and not humans on the most part.

In general terms, water fasting is simply a period when a person eats no food, take no beverage and drinks only water. For a healthy body and also for weight loss, this fast is effective. As regards the longevity of its effectiveness, there is a still a big question mark hanging over it. While it can and has actually helped some people lose weight in the short-term, it is factually not a suitable long term approach to health or weight loss or the likes of these, and it sets you on a course of risk, risk for health complications.

Other benefits of water fast as we shall see in detail shortly include lowering the risk of some chronic diseases and stimulating autophagy. No matter the reason that is selected as the goal for embarking on water fast, it is important to make sure that water fasting is made safely; preparation and proper planning must be paramount, the timing for the fast must coincide with a period when energy will be expended less. Water fasting is quite popular but you should come within reach of actually doing it with prudence.

3.2   WHAT IS WATER FASTING?

As the name implies, it is a fast that requires abstention from every other thing, water been the only exception. This exclusion of every other thing covers any and all forms of beverages be they alcoholic or not. In simple terms, there should be no food. One of the primary goals of water fast is body cleansing. There are a couple of other cleansing models that have used the water fast as yardstick. For some of these, you will be required to stay on a water regulated regimen for upwards of 40 days.

For a majority of history, fasting has been for either religious obligation or for spiritual reasons be they cleansing, purification or deprivation. In our present day, fasting goes for reasons ranging from weight loss, good health, spiritual or religious obligations and the likes. Alongside meditation, fasting has become a veritable tool in the hands of the proponents of the natural health and wellness movements.

We have said that water fasting is a type of fast wherein you are not allowed to consume anything besides water and the duration of this is not set on stone but it is advised that on the average the minimum duration of water fast should not go below 24 hours and should not exceed the 72 hour mark. Any attempt to go outside or exceed this set duration must be strictly under medical supervision.

3.3   HOW TO WATER FAST

There are so many things in life that are simple in themselves but they are not easy to do. Water fast falls squarely under this category. The rule to abstain from food and beverage is simple but the ease of just consuming water alone is not a walk in the park. If you embark on water fast, it is advisable that you drink at the least two liters of water per day, but ideally this isn't up to speed as your body requires more than that since our water source also extends to food. So not eating food, you must account for the shortage in your water intake. For the first time, the sudden urge for more and more water must be hardly bearable or out rightly overwhelming so if you are doing a water fast for the first time, be sure to gradually condition your body by slowly cutting down your calorie consumption for a few days leading up to your fast.

At the close of water fast, make sure at least on the first day to resist the urge to splurge at a big meal. Whole scale digestive discomfort like constipation and bloating accompany the consumption of big meals especially right after restricting yourself from calories for an extended period of time. While it is unlikely, it possible that you will be at risk for re-feeding syndrome, a potentially grave condition that involves quick metabolic adjustments, usually in people who are extremely malnourished. Instead, give yourself a three day recovering period; begin by adding caloric beverages like milk or juice, on the second day carefully introduce snacks and small meals. When the third day comes round, you should be able to eat normally again.

Since it is simple, there are no strict guidelines on how to begin water fasting. This simplicity nevertheless, there exist persons who first water fasting is not suited for or persons should not water fast without medical supervision. This includes people diagnosed diabetes or gout, people with eating disorders, pregnant women and children, and older adults. For people who want to attempt the water fast for the very first time, however there is a rule: spend three to four days preparing your body for being without food. You can get your body prepared by either eating smaller portions consecutively at each meal or by fasting for part of the day.

The water fast is simple but no doubt not easy since it is the most grueling type of fast. A word of warning is necessary here. The tempting part to water fast is the fact that water fast costs nothing to do, but can lead to major gains such as weight loss, focus on your inner spiritual life, and possibly the flushing out of toxins from the body. As a result we can get carried away. While is true that every attempt at short-term calorie restriction does help make life longer and healthier especially when done correctly, we must noted that fasting can also be dangerous. Whatever your reason, drive, intention or goal, advance into water fasting safely – take time to bask in it, recognize signs of when to stop, and transition back to food slowly. In all you do, carry a qualified medical professional along.

3.4 PLANNING YOUR WATER FAST

Know your medical state. Ignorance of your medical state and possible medical conditions can lead to a breakdown or worsening when you fast. This has been shown to lead to serious health consequences. Water fast is advisably off limits to you if you suffer from any of the following:

- Lupus
- Paralysis
- Alcoholism
- Post-transplant
- Late stage cancer

- Enzyme deficiency
- Thyroid dysfunction
- Live long medication
- Pregnant or breastfeeding
- Any eating disorder e.g. anorexia
- Late stage kidney or liver disease
- Vascular disease or poor circulation
- AIDS, tuberculosis, or infectious disease
- Low blood sugar (hypoglycemia) or diabetes
- Alzheimer's disease or organic brain syndrome
- Heart disease, including heart failure, or history of a heart attack

Select duration. To start, try something short, that is, a 1-day water fast. Prudence and experience require that you limit your water fast to three days if you are not under supervision or guidance. Studies and personal observation suggests that just on an average, a one to three day short-term fast can have the best health benefits. If you plan on fasting longer than that, ensure that you get medical supervision. It is rather safer and may offer more health benefits to fast for short times periodically, rather than doing a five or one week long fast. You might even take into consideration, the possibility of doing water fast for two days out of the week at the most.

Find a low-stress time. Water fast must always come at the best possible time for the best results so be careful that your water fast is planned for when your stress levels will be minimal. This is best when fasting will not interfere markedly with your daily routine. As much as will be possible, ensure you keep away from working while fasting. Target your rest corridors; situate your fast within a time frame that allows you rest both physically and mentally.

Prepare mentally. We have stressed the fact that fasting for multiple days can be daunting. Thought of it is also mentally tasking. Hence, you can prepare but having a chat with your doctor, read books on the subject such as this one, and reaching out to other people you know who have fasted. Look up to the actual fast as you would an adventure.

Switch to your fast mode. Your body will better welcome and contain the fast when you dig into it gradually so you must start small. Switch into your fast mode by eliminating sugar, processed foods, and even caffeine from your diet progressively least 2-3 days before your fast. In the place of what you eliminate, consume generous amounts of fruits and vegetables. The size of your meals must reduce progressively leading up to your fast. Consider skipping breakfast or/and lunch and decreasing your portion for dinner intermittently till you begin your water fast.

3.5   CARRYING OUT YOUR FAST

Drink plenty water. Since it is water fast, water is indispensible key to the success of this fast. You must set out a way to ensure that you drink on the average three liters of water a day. You must be careful to stay within this recommended amount so as not to throw off the salt/mineral balance in your body. Drink water in batches and make sure to space it evenly. Choose water sources that are clean so as not to cause health problems for you.

Handling hunger. Since you have trained your body with the habit of eating when hunger pangs set it, hunger pangs will definitely come periodically. Here you must rewire the habit, drink couple of glasses of water through the pangs and try to distract yourself when the pangs persist. You can try activities that require less energy such as meditation, reading or even sleeping. Be sure to rest.

Breaking fast. When the time comes round for you to break your fast, do so slowly and gradually. You can begin with juice then little chunks of food a few hours apart. Spread your eating time evenly to match your fast duration. Be sure to eat the heavy foods only a couple of days after.

3.6 POTENTIAL BENEFITS OF WATER FASTING

There are promising potential benefits of water fasting, but it's important to note that research on the benefits of water fast are all agreeing on the endless benefits such fast without ample cases of reference to humans. This is not limiting as such research are ongoing. This shortcoming notwithstanding, Amanda Capritto & Claire Sissons have graciously delineated a few benefits. Endless benefits of water fasting succinctly include;

- Lowers blood pressure
- Encourages Better Insulin Sensitivity
- Lowers the risk of several chronic diseases
- Promotes weight loss
- Improves Cell Recycling
- Protects against diabetes
- Improves Body Composition and Fitness
- Protects Your Brain
- Promotes Heart Health

- Decreases Inflammation
- Promotes Greater Satiety
- Boosts Your Metabolism
- Improves Blood Triglycerides
- Supports Fat Loss and Ketosis
- Improves Cardiovascular Health
- Supports Healthier Collagen in Skin
- Reduces Harmful Protein Production
- Promotes a Healthy Stress Response
- Increases Resistance to Oxidative Stress
- May Slow Aging and Enhance Longevity

Let us elaborate on a few of these health benefits below.

3.6.1 May Lower Blood Pressure

High salt intake and poor water consumption are two clear factors that lead to higher blood pressures and a reverse of these will lower blood pressure readings. This reversal is achievable with the help of the water fast. It is a veritable tool to manage blood pressure.

3.6.2 Encourages better Insulin Sensitivity

Hormones such as Insulin together with leptin greatly affect body metabolism. These hormones have distinct functions in the body. While insulin aids the body store nutrients from the food in the bloodstream, leptin one the other hand enables the body feel full. The functioning of these two hormones become more apt upon water fasting. The result of this aptness is greater sensitivity and more effectiveness. For example, with better insulin sensitivity your body is less prone to diabetes. Increased leptin sensitivity makes you more in control of handling hunger pangs which enables you to better lower the risk of ever become obese.

3.6.3 Lowers the Risk of Several Chronic Diseases

There is a possible connection that exists between water fast and the prevention of cancer or heart disease. At the end of the fast, your body will most definitely have lower levels of triglycerides and cholesterol, and these factors are wholly responsible for the outbreak of cardiovascular disease. Water fast will help reduce the growth of tumors it is believed. This has only been proven in animals in the meantime. There is some evidence that water fasting may lower the risk of chronic diseases like diabetes because of the increase in sensitivity of insulin after a water fast.

3.6.4 It Promotes Weight Loss

When the body is denied a constant supply of

carbs, which is the first port of call for energy, it reverts to fats. So, when on a water fast, the body is denied a steady supply of carbs (glucose and glycogen) it turns to fats, it supplies the body with much needed energy and reduces the possibility of becoming over weight. Water fast enables the body to use up the excess fats in the body and promote weight loss. When water fast can be done with regularity and combined with regular light exercise, the results on weight loss are better.

3.6.5 Improves Cell Recycling

The mechanisms at work within the human body are remarkably efficient. For instance, body cells are broken down and recycled daily following a mechanism autophagy. Primarily it widely accepted that it is through autophagy that cancer prevention can be enhanced. The effectiveness of this extends to the prevention of heart disease and Alzheimer's disease as well.

3.6.6 Protect Against Diabetes

Diabetes and insulin are linked. A rise in diabetes is a sign of insulin deficiency and vice versa. Now it has been demonstrated from countless study that fasting of any type can help to improve insulin sensitivity. Without a doubt, insulin resistance is the main factor in the development of diabetes, so when the body endures water fast insulin sensitivity is greatly enhanced and the risk of diabetes especially type 2 is decreased.

3.6.7 Improves body composition and fitness

Many people have imbalanced body composition as a result of poor dieting or over consumption of particular foods. This invariable wreaks their fitness levels leading to poor self esteem. With water fast issues such as inability to climb a flight stairs, endure exercise regimes and the likes are no more as the water level in the body reach optimal levels and improves fitness.

3.7 DANGERS AND RISKS OF WATER FASTING

Although water fasting has been demonstrated to have many benefits, it has its down sides as well. It is important to be watchful and conscious of the following before, while and after any duration of water fast. The benefits might be blinding such that we are tempted to cast a closed eye at the outset of any dangers or risks. Let us consider some these.

3.7.1 Losing the Wrong Type of Weight

People often talk about weight loss but hardly talk about the specific type of weight. It is a given that when you do a water fast you will lose weight but which weight you lose depends on your body make, diet pattern, etc. weight that can be lost include, excess fat, stored up carbs or even muscle mass. During water fast you lose weight rapidly to the tune of about five or six pounds after a three day fast. Care should be taken then to lose the right type of fat and not suffer because of wrong targeting.

3.7.2 Excessive Dehydration

It must sound counter intuitive to say that there is the chance of a person who is on a water fast suffering from dehydration. Odd as this might seem, it is true and remarkably possible because while it the case that you drink water during water fast, you can drink short of the required amount and be at risk for dehydration. A whole lot of the water we consume is not tabulated or recorded. So cutting away food also implies cutting away a water source and replacing this source by drinking water directly often falls short. So water fast could make you dehydrated. With dehydration come headaches, constipation, and low pressure in the blood. To counter this, we might fall into over hydration.

3.7.3 Orthostatic Hypotension

Orthostatic hypotension is a decrease in blood pressure that is occasioned when you suddenly rise from reclined position. The resultant feeling a few seconds upon rising usually makes you lightheaded and this condition is typical among people who water fast. When you experience orthostatic hypotension while you fast, then this fast may not be for you and to prevent incidence of accidents then there is the need to be more cautious of activity you involve yourself with while fasting.

3.7.4 Worsen Medical Conditions

Usually water fast lasts just three days at a time and within this brief time there are so many things that go wrong. Among these things are medical conditions such as gout which is aggravated by the increase in uric acid that water fast instigates, diabetes whose side effects can be heightened by water fast, eating disorders such as bulimia and anorexia, heartburn since the body will not have food to digest with the stomach acid present in the stomach.

3.7.5 Nutrient Deficiencies

It is easy to assume that it is just food that the body needs and it can go a couple of days without it. But hidden behind this assumption is the fact that there a number of essential elements that come with food intake and these include whole gamut of essential vitamins, minerals, fatty acids, amino acids, and electrolytes. The body requires all that to function properly and the source of such is through food intake. Water fasting good as it may seem might rob you of much needed nutrients.

3.7.6 Hyponatremia

Hyponatremia is a condition that occurs when saline fluids are lost and are replaced by water only. Hyponatremia happens usually when we sweat. This loss happens when we fast from food and beverage which ordinarily replace the needed salts. It is for this very reason that exercise and energy exerting task during water fast are not recommended. For persons who sweat a lot, this problem will be more troubling.

3.7.7 Trouble Focusing

It is generally recommended that less activity is carried out during water fast. The best periods for water fast are moments when we would be able to rest and refrain from strenuous work. This optimal state is difficult for many to come by in our rather frantic world. Persons who might need to go to work or school necessarily and still want to embark on water fast while at those activities should be ready for the trouble of fatigue and focusing. Mild–to-severe headaches and disorientations might be common to such people at such periods.

3.7.8 Binge Eating

Fasting frequently leads to binge eating. Binge eating is an eating disorder that is defined as the act of repeatedly eating indiscriminately out of obsession and not just for nutrition. While many people fast, they mentally think and fantasize about food and when they break their fast, there is the urge to splurge in a bit to gratify this craving.

3.8   SAFETY TIPS

It seems then that the possibility of falling into some danger or been at risk while you water fast far outweighs the benefits. In actuality this is not the case. Prudence however is advised and to be on the safe side, some tips are here provided to stem the events of risks or exposure to dangers native to water fast.

Ensure that you eat a healthy diet habitually. Many people often have eating disorders or are careless about their diet both in content and timing. They hope then that fasting will help correct their health or weight issues. There is hardly as way by which fating will help if prior to and after water fast if you eat haphazardly. To get the best our water fasting, make sure to follow a diet high in fruits, vegetables, and whole grains, and low in high/bad fats and high/refined sugar.

Ensure you exercise regularly. The importance of exercise to our bodies cannot be overstressed. When we exercise, we burn bad calories, sweat, our heart beat stabilizes and our muscles are toned among other things. Exercise for at least 30 minutes five days a week. This can be a brisk walk, light jogging, bike riding, running the treadmill or even something more engaging. Live a healthy daily life to perk up your physical condition and wellbeing, and fasting will be of more help to achieving this goal.

Consult your healthcare provider. Consult your healthcare provider when you are considering fasting. Fasting, as good as it is in itself, is not for everyone. For it will benefit some and be dangerous to others. Your healthcare provider is in the best place to determine how and when water fast would suit you. Though fasting may offer health benefits for some people, others should avoid it. Be sure to discuss your medications and medical conditions with your doctor to determine if water fasting is safe for you. This tip is all the more significant if you have a known health challenge or you are under medication.

Guarantee against dizziness. Dizziness may set in after a day into your fast and even after you break the fast. This will occur especially when you stand up quickly and to counter this get up slowly after some deep breathing. If you do get up and still get dizzy, immediately sit for awhile and if this continues, see you health care provider.

Get plenty of rest during your water fast. Rest is crucial during water fast and do all you can to respect it. Ensure to engage in activities such as light reading, meditation, napping and do not overexert yourself by any means. Be on a low key physically. Avoid exercise that are exerting during fasting. Yoga is permissible. Listen raptly to your body and only get something done that feels comfortable.

Get your timing right. Fasting for longer than 3 days requires prior planning. It is advised to do a one day trial first and evaluate how it went. The weekend or when on leave is best. There can be no better time to put fasting than in comfort of your home while resting.

Plan well ahead. Nothing can substitute for a good plan made well ahead. The possible pitfalls, challenges and nuances are all worked out and measures set to handle them. A to-do list should be made while planning for the fast and every item should be addressed well ahead of the intended fasting period. For instance, eating healthy days before the fast, pick the best time that will allow for optimum rest, getting materials to read, selecting out yoga exercise patterns, ensuring availability of a good water source, seeing the doctor for tests and advice, plan feeding patterns for after the fast.

3.9   QUESTIONS ON WATER FAST

1. Will Water Fasting Help You Burn Fat?

Yes, water fasting can help you burn fat but if this is your sole reason for wanting to fast, water fast would not be that effective on the long term. On the long term, water fast will help you lose more of water, carbs and muscle mass than fats. Other forms of fasting such as intermittent fasting and alternate day fasting regimes would be better suited to achieve that goal. Read up the parts that we discussed the other forms of fast to see what would be best suited for your goal.

2. Who should not fast?

Fasting is a good practice but it not for everyone. Certain categories of people should not fast and if they must, they must seek professional guidance from qualified persons. These people who are exempt include the elderly, children under 15, special persons (persons have an eating disorder, have uncontrolled migraines, are pregnant or breast-feeding, are undergoing a blood transfusion, have heart problems, have type 1 diabetes, are underweight, and are taking specific medication). Note that this list is not by any means exhaustive.

3 Is water fasting any safer if you still have a lot of body fat to lose?

Body size is not the adequate measure of body fat. Our body makeup is also fat based.

Structural protein for example are the basic building blocks of your muscle mass, which means that your body might be eating itself away rather eating up what is assumed to be excess fat.

4. Is water fasting safe at all?

Yes it is safe and advisable. Seek the consent and advice of a healthcare provider before embarking on it and ensure to keep your fasts short (preferably under 72 hours, that is, three consecutive days at most), space the timing in between your fasts (minimum of two weeks apart), and consider safer fasting alternatives (intermittent fasting and alternate day fasting).

5. How much water should I drink during my water fast?

The human body is water based and requires water to function properly. In fact about 60% of our body is plainly water. The need to drink water cannot be over stressed. It is necessary then to drink enough quantity of water daily, this amount varies from fasting and unfasting states. While fasting the glasses should be 12 and 14 for men and between 8 and 10 for females. Three liters should be the golden mean at all times.

6. How long can a person water fast?

It should be at least three days at a time and a minimum of two weeks in between the fasts. There is the temptation to extend the days when you feel comfortable but this must be resisted so that it does not become habitual.

7. Who can benefit from water fasting?

There are ample benefits for anyone who is able to do a water fast.

PART FOUR: GENERAL FASTING TYPES

4.1   INTRODUCTION

Within this part we shall dwell upon the religious dimension or way of fasting. We shall try to be very eclectic and touch upon most of the major world religions with careful attention to the nuances that exists among the different religions or sects. From the religious angle, fasting is largely observed as a fulfillment of religious obligation or for spiritual purposes. We shall look at the Baha'I faith, Buddhism, Christianity (Roman Catholicism, Eastern Orthodoxy, Lutheranism, and Pentecostalism), Hinduism, Islam and Judaism.

4.2   RELIGIOUS FASTS

Religious fasts as the name suggests are done for spiritual, religious or ritual reasons. For instance, the Daniel Fast is reproduction model following the book of Daniel in the Bible. This is a type of partial fast putting a ceiling on all foods except all fruits, some vegetables, grains and water for 21 days. In another case, the Jewish Tzomot is known to include seven diverse religious fasts through the course of the calendar year. Ramadan is an Islamic fast, lasting one month (this can be consequent 30 days or with breaks but eventually totaling 30 days) during which Muslims fast from break of day to end of the day. More specifically, let us look at fasting within the world's major religions.

4.3   BAHÁ'Í

For Bahá'í Faith adherents, Bahá'u'lláh outlined the rule in the Kitáb-i-Aqdas that fasting is customarily observed from break of day to sundown during the Bahá'í month of 'Ala' which corresponds roughly to 1 or 2 March – 19 or 20 March. This fast complete. It entails total abstention from both food and drink during daylight hours. While this abstention extends to smoking, it gives ample room for any consumption of prescribed medications at any time of the day it may be required. Observing the fast is an individual obligation and is binding on Bahá'ís between their official year of maturity (15 years) and 70 years old. As a result to be exempted from this mandating principle one had to be younger than the official maturity age or have celebrated his 70th birthday. Other exceptions to the fasting requirements are those under the pain of illness; women who are menstruating, pregnant, or nursing; adherents whose line of work involves intense labor and those who are naturally frail or very sick, for whom fasting would ordinarily not be safe. For those occupied in jobs with serious labor, it is recommended that they, while they eat out of necessity, do so in private and in general restrict themselves to smaller meals than are normal. Fasting, according to this faith, reinvigorates the spiritual forces latent in the soul. It's worth and rationale are, necessarily, fundamentally spiritual in character and symbolic. Fasting ultimately is a reminder of abstinence from selfish and carnal desires.

4.4   BUDDHISM

Fasting is carried out by lay Buddhists within their times of thorough meditation, for instance, during a retreat. During periods of fasting, adherents of Buddhism completely keep away from consuming animal products, although allowance is made for the consumption of milk. Moreover, they also prohibit the consumption of processed foods and the five pungent foods which are; garlic, garlic chives, asana, welsh onion, leeks. The Middle Path refers to avoiding any possible crossing of the boundaries of indulgence on the one hand and self-mortification on the other. Buddhist monks and nuns following the Vinaya rules generally do not eat each day after the noon meal. This is not regarded a fast but rather a regimented regimen designed to foster meditation and good health.

4.5   CHRISTIANITY

Fasting, as an obligation or voluntary act, is an inherent tradition in a number of Christian sects. It is customarily observed both on a collective basis during certain seasons of the liturgical calendar, or on an individual level as a believer feel inspired by the Holy Spirit.

Now in the long history of Western Christianity, fast is most revered and observed particularly during the Lenten season by many baptized of the Catholic Church first, then those of the Reformed

Churches, Methodists, Lutherans, those   of the Western Orthodox Churches, and of the Anglican Communion. This fast is gradually extending to the protestants, although they do not call it the Lenten fast, they generally observe it around the same time as the other churches do.

This Lenten fast is a forty-day partial fast in remembrance of the fast carried out by Christ before his temptation in the desert. While some Western Christians observe the Lenten fast wholly, only the duo of Ash Wednesday (the beginning of Lent) and Good

Friday (at the close of Lent) are in this day and age emphasized by Roman Catholicism as the normative days of fasting within the Lenten season. Then there is the traditional Black Fast in which the observant abstains from food for a whole day in anticipation of the evening, and at day's end, traditionally breaks the fast.

Roman Catholicism

Fasting is obligatory for the faithful between the ages of 18 and 59 on particular days. Within catholic tradition, fasting, considered as a native jargon, is the conscious and deliberate lessening of one's intake of food to one full meal. More specifically, this fast must not contain meat on Ash Wednesday, Good Friday, and Fridays throughout the entire Lenten season and may continue throughout the year. Then two small meals which in liturgical terminology is collation, both meals are taken one in the daybreak and the other in the late afternoon of which together should not equal the large meal. Eating solid food between meals is prohibited.

In addition to the fasts mentioned above, Roman Catholics must also observe the Eucharistic Fast, which involves taking nothing except water and medicines into the body for one hour before receiving the

Eucharist.

Eastern Orthodoxy

For Eastern Orthodox Christians, from both the Old Testament and the New, fasting is an important spiritual discipline, and it has been found to be tied to the principle in Orthodox theology on the synergy between the body and the soul. In Eastern Orthodoxy, fasting can take up a noteworthy part of the calendar year. According to Sacred Tradition, the rationale of fasting is to guard against gluttony and impure thoughts, deeds and words not to suffer. For them, fasting must all the time be accompanied by better prayer and almsgiving, donating to a local charity, general philanthropy or directly to the poor, depending on the state of affairs.

Lutheranism

The Protestant Reformer, Martin Luther, is claimed to have held that fasting served to "kill and subdue the pride and lust of the flesh". As a result of the forgoing claim, the Lutheran churches often emphasized voluntary fasting over collective fasting, despite the fact that certain liturgical seasons and holy days were times for communal fasting and abstinence. This position has spread out far into the Pentecostal movement. These days it is hardly possible ascertain for the pattern this claim has used to infiltrate the Christian world.

Pentecostalism

Even though Pentecostalism has not classified different types of fasting, certain pastors or church leaders within the movement have done so. So there are different shades and days for fasting according to the inspiration or direction of the pastors. So it is safe to conclude then that Pentecostalism as generally known does not have set days of abstinence, but individuals in the movement may feel they are being directed by the Holy Spirit to undertake either short or extended fasts often times when they are about to or while asking God for a favour or blessing. Abstinence from food is also encouraged with supporting biblical verses for members any time they yearn to grow nearer to God and to put into effect self-mastery of spirit over body. Those who follow the movement may also put into practice family, group or even personal, fasts any time they aspire to importune special blessings from God, this can include health or prosperity or comfort for themselves or others.

4.6   HINDUISM

Individuals observe different kinds of fasts based on personal beliefs and local customs. Abstinence is a very central part of the Hindu religion. Some Hindus fast on certain days of the month such as Ekadasi, or Pradosha. Personal belief and favorite deity are reasons that determine the way certain days of the week are also set aside for fasting. For instance, Tuesday fasting is widespread in southern India as well as northwestern India but Thursday fasting is common among the Hindus of northern India. These special fasts extend to fasting during religious festivals as this practice is also very common. For the Hindus, methods of fasting vary widely and, in addition to the above instances, cover a broad spectrum. If in its strictest form, the person fasting does not involve himself in the consumption of any food or water from the previous day's sunset until 48 minutes after the following day's sunrise. Hindus also claim that when you fast you limit yourself to one meal during the day, eating only or abstaining from eating certain food types.

4.7   ISLAM

Muslims believe like the Catholics that fasting is a lot more than abstaining from just food and drink. It also entails abstaining from any lying, misleading or deceit, abstaining from any speech that is indecent or non edifying, and from all forms of arguing, physical assault or fight, and having lustful thoughts. The essence of all these is that in the end fasting is supposed to have strengthened control of impulses and generally lent a hand to the development of good behavior. During Ramadan, fasting is obligatory for every Muslim and this is observed one month in the year. Each day, the fast begins at dawn and ends at sunset. Similar exceptions are given in consideration for classes of people who will be adversely affected just as, children who are too young; Serious illness that require strong medications; A woman during her menstrual period; A woman who is pregnant or breast feeding among others are not required to fast.

4.8 JUDAISM

Fasting for Jews is simple; it entails absolute abstinence from food and drink, including water. There are no ways around it. It is either one is observing the fast or not. It is expected for every devout Jew fast six days of the year. Fasting is never permitted on Shabbat, except for the feast of Yom Kippur, for the commandment of keeping Shabbat is biblically ordained and supersedes the later rabbinically instituted fast days. For reasons of seeking repentance in the event of tragedy or some imminent misfortune Aside from these official days of fasting, Jews may take upon themselves personal or communal fasts,. In the time of the Talmud, drought seems to have been a particularly frequent inspiration for fasts.

PART FIVE – INTERMITTENT FAST

5.1   INTRODUCTION

Within this part, we shall dwell intensively upon intermittent fasting. This form of fast as we shall see later is not a form of dieting rather it is a pattern of eating. Thereafter we shall succinctly, fix our focus on the alternates of the fed and fasted states. An understanding of the dissimilarity between these states reveals the way by which this mode of fasting works. We have delineated seven types of intermittent fast. We shall dutifully explain the nature and procedure for: The 16/8 Method, The 5:2 Diet, The Eat-Stop-Eat, The Alternate Day Fasting, The Warrior Diet, The Spontaneous Meal Skipping, and The Daily Intermittent Fast.

Sequel to this we shall dwell upon the procedure of carrying out intermittent fast. They are goal identification, method selection, specification of calorie needs, setting out meal plans and making calories count in that order.

The two things left to deal with on intermittent fast is the benefits and side effects. First, we shall generally list out the factors that will increase, those that will decrease and those factors that will improve. Only after this will the particular benefits such as the ability of intermittent fast to make our days simpler, add years to our lives, free us from the clutches of cancer and make our diets easier. While the cloud of intermittent fast has its silver lining, it has its backsides. The side effects we shall look at include and is limited to fatigue, hunger, binger eating, dehydration and tiredness.

5.2   WHAT IS INTERMITTENT FAST?

Intermittent fasting is often mistaken to be a form of dieting, it is not a diet; it is a pattern of eating. It is a pattern of eating because fundamentally, it is a way of scheduling the meals you eat in order that you get the largest part out of them. In other words, it is right to claim that intermittent fasting does not modify *what* you eat, it alters *when* you eat. Why is it meaningful to amend when you eat? Well, most markedly, it is a striking way to acquire a lean physique without going on an extreme diet or slashing your calories down to zilch. For a large part of the time you could be able to maintain your calorie count at a stable rate when you launch intermittent fasting because a good number people eat larger meals during a shorter time framework. Furthermore, intermittent fasting is a high-quality way to maintain muscle mass on a steady rate while getting slender.

There is no gainsaying that the most important reason people try intermittent fasting is to shake off fat. It is necessary then to consider how intermittent fasting leads to fat loss more specifically. Rather pertinently, intermittent fasting is one of the simplest stratagem generally available taking harmful weight off while maintaining healthy weight on simply on the reason that it requires quite modest behavior amendment. This is an exceptionally excellent thing because it signifies that intermittent fasting falls into the class of straightforward and easy that you will most easily do it, but remarkably meaningful enough that the difference it makes will become visible.

5.3   HOW INTERMITTENT FASTING WORKS

To have a full grasp of how intermittent fasting

brings about fat loss we foremost need to comprehend the dissimilarity between the two states we often alternate between; the fed state and the fasted state. Let me explain these states in simple terms, your body is considered to be in the fed state at what time it is breaking down and absorbing food. Characteristically, the fed state kicks off the moment you commence eating and continues for upwards of five hours as your body digests and sucks up the food you just consumed. Following that time duration, your body enters what is regarded as the post–absorptive state, which is just a flowery manner of saying that your body is not processing a meal. Note that because your insulin levels are elevated at the time that you are in the fed state, it is very difficult for your body to breakdown fat. You enter the fasted state 8 to 12 hours after your last meal because after these hours you body is outside the absorbing stage. Your insulin levels are low in the fasted state and it is much trouble-free for your body to burn fat.

Your body can not burn fat in your fed state because many of the fat is simply inaccessible but such fats become accessible when you are in the fasted state. Recall that I explained above that it is not until the twelfth hour after our last meal that we enter the fasted state. This corroborates the assertion I made on the fact that it is not what we eat but when we eat that determines the rate of fat that our body burns. This is another of the reasons that explains why a large number of people who observe intermittent fasting will lose fat without altering the contents of their food, the amount of food they consume, or how often they exercise. Fasting locks your body in a fat burning state that you hardly ever get into during a normal eating program.

5.4   TYPES OF INTERMITTENT FAST

1. The 16/8 Method.
This method tends to follow a natural pattern. This method made prevalent by the fitness expert Martin Berkhan is also branded as the Leangains practice. For majority of persons who find themselves hungry in the morning and are accustomed to eat breakfast, then this

can be rather tough to get adapted to at inception. Embarking upon this scheme of fasting can in reality be as simple as maintaining the hunger state till the break of day, and skipping breakfast. For example, after you must have had your dinner within the traditional 6-8pm time frame and then you don't eat until about noon the following day, then in principle you are already fasting for 16 hours between your last meal and subsequent meals. However, many breakfast skippers actually instinctively eat this way. In essence then, the 16/8 Method comprises fasting daily for a minimum of 14 and maximum of 16 hours, and making sure to confine your daily eating period to a minimum of 8 and maximum of 10 hours. Within the eating period, it is permissible to fit in 2 or more meals. For women the fasting duration is slightly shorter for it is strongly suggested that women only fast 14-15 hours, the guiding principle behind this exception is the discovery that they seem to achieve superior results with somewhat shorter fasts.

We have said that the 16/8 method involves

daily fasts of 16 hours for men, and a slightly shorter duration for women. Likewise we carefully explained that on each day, it mandatory to confine your eating to an 8-10 eating hour period. It is quite important to stick to eating largely healthy foods while within you eating period. This fasting method will not work or achieve much for you if you consume junk food regularly or in excess or you focus on taking in disproportionate amounts of calories. In order to keep hunger levels at the barest minimum during the fasting window then, you can drink coffee without milk, water, and other non-caloric beverages. Personally, I consider this to be the only way that is mainly close to the natural way to do intermittent fasting. I follow this regimen myself and find it to be perfectly effortless. Since I stick to a diet that is majorly low-carb, my appetite is dulled to a large extent. The result is that I usually hardly until around 1 pm in the afternoon the next day and because stick to having my last meal around 6-9 pm, I end up fasting for upwards of 16-19 hours.

2. The 5:2 Diet.

There are seven days in a week and of these full seven days, this type of intermittent fasting requires that special attention is paid to two days out of the seven. So in essence, the 5:2 method of fasting or dieting is one that requires two days within the week which should not be consecutive days be set aside for limited calorie intake. Calorie intake on these selected days should not exceed 500-600. For instance, you might choose to eat as is normal for you on all days of the week except on say Tuesdays and Fridays, on which days you eat two small meals totaling but not exceeding 300 calories per meal for men and 250 calories for women. Hence on each fasting day calorie intake does not exceed 500 for women and 600 for men. The British Journalist and Doctor, Michael Mosley is credited with popularizing this form of intermittent fasting which is a form of diet and is called the Fast diet. While there is no denying that there are plenty of studies on the benefits of intermittent fasting, critics are right to insist that there is a dearth of literature and experiments on the efficacy of this form of intermittent fasting.

3. Eat-Stop-Eat.

This form of fast in close to the 5:2 diet method of intermittent fast, only that in this method there is complete fast for full twenty four hours. This can be repeated on two or three days within the same week but care should be taken so as not to fast on two consecutive days within the same week. This twenty four hour fast can be taken in either of three ways, which is from breakfast to breakfast, lunch to lunch or dinner to dinner. The most common of the three is often the dinner to dinner fast. So if you take your dinner on Tuesday by 6pm and only eat again by 6pm on Wednesday, you would have fasted successfully for twenty four hours. Whichever duration is chosen, the result is always the same. While in the 5:2 fast calorie intake was restricted, the eat-stop-eat only permits intakes of water, coffee and other non-caloric beverages during the fast, but on no account should solid food be taken. This method which has been quite popular for a few years has been championed by fitness expert Brad Pilon. Many people who chose this method are often aiming at losing weight, for such persons it is necessary that during their eating cycles they eat normally without restrictions or dieting. The fasting cycles help the body meet with the weight loss goals. The only drawback is the very strong craving that hits you during the last few hours of the fast. Many people find handling this urge very difficult or even near to impossible. The best way to deal with this challenge is begin with a 16 hour cycle then gradually increase the hours at subsequent attempts.

4. Alternate-Day Fasting.

Alternate-day fasting denotes fasting every other day. This can be achieved either by not eating anything or restricting eating to only a few hundred calories during the fasting days. Alternate-Day fasting portends a continuous cycle of fasting every other day for a couple of weeks. There are several different versions of this. Some versions make allowance for intake of about 500 calories during the fasting days.

Many other versions simply warrant the observance of complete dry fast. The version that requires full and complete dry fast can be a long shot for beginners. In itself it appears extreme. Hence this is not recommended for people who are just beginners as the adverse effects might bring about unwanted results. With this routine, it is clear that you will have to go to bed very famished three to four times per week, which is not very agreeable and almost certainly untenable in the long-standing. The good news is that whichever the version, studies have shown several health benefits of intermittent fasting.

5. The Warrior Diet.

The Warrior Diet has arguably been considered one of the foremost fasting regimes or diets that include a variety of intermittent fasting. It is common among people targeting fitness because in essence, the Warrior Diet focuses on what is eaten within each day. While there is provision for a huge meal at dinner time, restrictions come to fore during the day with allowances only for fruits and vegetables. The chief proponent of the Warrior Diet is the acclaimed fitness expert Ori Hofmekler. Following his description, it involves eating small amounts of raw fruits and vegetables during the day, then eating one huge meal at night. Basically, he explains that you are required to fast all day and feast heartily at night. This diet also gives emphasis to food selections that are of the composition as a paleo diet - entire, unprocessed foods that bear a close resemblance to their likes in nature.

6. Spontaneous Meal Skipping.

This form of fasting is the easiest regime to follow. It is simple and rule free. There is not any strict structure to follow yet there are a couple of benefits that can be reaped. This option simply requires that you skip meals from time to time at your pleasure; this can be when you do not feel hungry or when you are too occupied to cook and eat. Oftentimes while we are in transit or at work it is near impossible to find anything we want to eat, we are forced in such circumstances to do a short fast.

Skipping 1 or 2 meals when you feel so disposed is fundamentally a spontaneous intermittent fast. This form of fasting writes off the common myth that people must eat every few hours or they will become lean, loose muscle mass or even starve. The human body as constituted has been suited for the rigors of prolonged periods of famine, missing one or two meals from time to time does not cause damage or considerable harm to the body. For many of us, it is almost a tradition to daily skip breakfast and only eat a healthy lunch and dinner. Just make sure to eat healthy foods at the other meals. An added more innate way to do intermittent fasting is to plainly skip 1 or 2 meals when you do not feel hungry or do not have time to eat.

7. A Final Schedule of Intermittent Fasting: Daily Intermittent Fast

It is claimed in theory and practice that intermittent fasting could be the basis for weight loss, improvement in metabolic health and perhaps even extension of lifespan. It is therefore not in any way astonishing given the reputation that several different types/methods of intermittent fasting have been thought up. It is as a result of similar reasons as these that intermittent fasting has been very trendy in recent years. All of them can be effective, but which one fits best will depend on the individual. If you are making an allowance for trying out fasting, there are a number of diverse options for working it into your lifestyle. More generally, it is possible to reduce the types we have seen above to just three expansive forms of intermittent fasting. Let us expand upon the most common which is the daily intermittent fast.

For the most part of the time, the Leangains model of intermittent fasting is more followed. Recall that this model uses a 16–hour fast followed by an 8–hour eating period. Two things are attributed to Martin Berkhan first is the fact that he made this model of daily intermittent fasting trendy and secondly it is by him that the name originated.

Repetitions and practice of routines soon becomes habit and second nature to us. Actions or pattern of actions that are carried out daily soon become habit. Now for the reason that daily intermittent fasting is practiced every single day it soon turns out to be very easy to get into the custom of eating on this plan. Inadvertently, we have trained our bodies into eating at specific times and we hardly think about this regular occurrence. We have become accustomed to this and it is now second nature. The same thing happens with daily intermittent fasting; you inadvertently become skilled at not eating at certain times, you will always do this effortlessly.

The time you elect to start your 8–hour eating period does not matter. It is possible to start from 9am and stop at 5pm. Just as it is also possible to kick off at 1pm and end at 10pm. While I will not recommend this second instance since eating late comes with attendant issues like bloating or constipation, you must in all things settle upon whatever works best for you. Without prejudice to your freedom and likes, I would personally recommend that you settle upon the 1pm to 8pm model because it gives you the advantage of missing out on lunch which work often prevents us from eating and allowing you the privilege of eating dinner with friends and family. For many persons breakfast is naturally a meal that we often skip without a second thought.

It is remarkably easy to fall into the habit of skipping a meal during the day and this holds many benefits for us but this tradition is not all positive, one prospective shortcoming of this plan is that it becomes more difficult especially at the onset to make up for the same number of calories in during the week. In simple terms, there is not shortcut to get accustomed to eating larger meals on a steady basis. This drawback is important to point here because the most visible sign of intermittent fasting is weight loss and this can be a bad thing for some people. Most persons who embark on this routine appreciate the effect it has on their weight but for some others it is not their goal hence, it is a setback.

The most basic thing to be on the lookout for is consistency for about 85% of the time no matter the types of intermittent fasting schedule chosen and a freedom to eat just about anything you settle upon the remaining 15% of the time. so when you are invited for an occasional dinner or a sit out, do well to feast as is required of the occasion. Note carefully that while the routine is there as guide, it is not a hard and fast rule to get enslaved to.

5.5   HOW TO INTERMITTENT FAST

There are salient points about intermittent fast that have been pointed out earlier on in this book and reiterated at subsequent times and for the sake of emphasis and clarity it is pertinent to recall the following details:

- Intermittent fasting is not strictly a diet.

- It is a time based regulation to eating.

- Intermittent fasting neither restricts calorie sources nor specifies what foods should be eaten or avoided.

- Intermittent fasting most specifically has the health benefit of weight loss.

- It is not a fasting routine that suitable for just about anyone.

- Intermittent fasting basically involves alternating using varying time regulations between periods of eating and fasting.

- At inception, the fasting stages may seem like forced starvation and the urge to eat will be stronger and more pressing. This eventually wanes.

- Apart from weight loss, intermittent fasting is a wide spread method that people use to simplify their life, improve their overall well-being.

The disclaimer on the suitability of fasting for everyone must also be pointed out here again. For healthy and well-nourished people fasting has been demonstrated through countless reviews to be safe and appropriate. The same cannot be said for persons with medical conditions, very young children and the aged, menstruating females. Those for whom fasting is inappropriate notwithstanding, the salient tips that follow help ensure that the right type of intermittent fast is settled upon and make the experience easy and worthwhile.

1. Identify Goals

Aristotle began his book on ethics with the proposition that every action is thought to aim at some good. As to what the good is, he went on to explain and develop. This good can be said to be the goal. Following this principle, the prologue to any activity must be goal setting; hence, naturally, a person who embarks upon intermittent fasting ought to have the good of such activity in mind. The goal then for anyone going aboard intermittent fast may vary from the need to lose weight, improve metabolic health, or improve overall health. A person's ultimate goal will help them determine the most suitable fasting method.

2. Choose Method

As pointed out severally before, the beginning is always very challenging especially in overcoming the urge to eat. In this regard, it is recommended that whatever method is settled upon, a person should stay glued to one fasting method for at least 21 days or three weeks before undertaking yet another.

Out of the eat-stop-eat, warrior diet, lean gains and alternate day fasting, a person may try any when fasting for health reasons. A person should pick the plan that suits their preferences and which they think they can stick with. Note that little tweaks can be made to any of the methods settled upon though care should be taken not to make whole scale changes.

3. Specify Calories Needs

A person could choose to speak to their healthcare provider or dietitian for tips on how many calories your lifestyle requires. When you set out to control your total calorie intake, you most likely end up taking in more calories on the long run. For any calorie based regulation that seeks to consume less energy than is used seems already skewed and would ordinarily lead to failure. But this is not so. People with the need to lose weight could do with creating a calorie deficit for themselves — what this means is that they must consume less energy than they actually use. People whose goal is to gain weight need to consume more calories than they use.

There are no dietary restrictions when doing intermittent fasting, but note that this does not mean that calories do not count. There are a couple of digital tools available to help a person work out, monitor or regulate their caloric needs and determine just about the right amount of calories they need to consume each day to either gain or lose weight.

4. Figure out Meal Plans

The method we select to follow has its meal timing schedule. The need then to figure out meal plans becomes imperative. Meal planning as a conscious activity places before us some riches one of which is maintenance of your calorie count. Meal planning ensures that ahead of time you have the necessary food on hand, picked out cooking recipes, solutions for quick meals, and a constant supply of snacks. It is clear then that as constraining as meal planning seems it does not need to be overly limiting. If properly done, it adequately considers calorie intake and incorporates suitable nutrients into the diet. Planning ahead for the week may help someone who is trying to lose or gain weight feel ready mentally and physically. There is not a doubt that anyone intent on shedding or putting on weight would discover the treasures of pre-planning what they are going to eat.

5. Make Calories Count

Calories are not all the same. This makes the need to make every calorie we consume count. The amount of calories we need to consume is not highly regulated by whatever fasting method we have chosen but it is quite necessary to always keep under careful consideration the nutritional value of all the food we take. This re-echoes the need for planning our meals. On a broad spectrum, during the eating phase of a fasting regime, it is all important to focus on consuming food with high nutrient density, foods that their nutrient per calorie ratio is high. This calls for moderation in intake of junk food as they are often not very healthy options. Sparse indulgence may not cause much harm and is acceptable.

5.6   BENEFITS OF INTERMITTENT FAST

We have pointed out a couple of times before now that the major benefit of intermittent fast is weight loss. It is general knowledge that fat loss is great especially excessive fat, there is no way this is the only benefit of fasting. More succinctly, the benefits are:

Factors that will decrease

- Intermittent fasting helps reduce blood lipids (including decreased triglycerides and LDL cholesterol)

- It moderates blood pressure (this is possible since it ensures changes in sympathetic/parasympathetic activity)

- It trims down indicators of inflammation (including CRP<, IL-6, TNF, BDNF, and more)

- It diminishes all instances of oxidative stress (using pointers of protein and DNA damage)

- It cuts down the risk of cancer (by means of a mass of projected mechanisms)

Factors that will increase

- Intermittent fasting helps in the proliferation of cellular turnover and repair (autophagocytosis)

- It intensifies fat burning (increase in intensity of fatty acid oxidation especially in the later stages of the fast)

- It multiplies growth hormone release in the latter stages of the fast (hormonally mediated)

- It boosts metabolic rate (this metabolic rate is stimulated by epinephrine and norepinephrine release)

The following will be improved

- chemotherapy effectiveness (by permitting elevated doses more regularly)
- appetite management (most likely through modifications in PPY and ghrelin)
- cardiovascular role (fortification against ischemic damage to the heart)
- blood sugar management (by moderating blood glucose and boosting insulin sensitivity)
- neuronal flexibility and neurogenesis (by ensuring defense against neurotoxins)

More broadly it has been demonstrated from countless studies and personal accounts that intermittent fasting can achieve the following added together:

1. Simpler Days.

Been in favor of behavior modification, simplicity, and stress reduction, intermittent fasting facilitates additional simplicity to the life of anyone who practices it and I can argue that that experience is wholly joy giving. Upon rising at the break of day there is hardly any need to become fretted about breakfast. The day can be kicked off with a simple glass of water. The only challenge here will be the need to miss the first meal of the day. The advantage been the reduced stress on cooking early in the day and rushing to eat before or after dressing up for work as the case may apply. The hassle of planning for meals is reduced by one as well as stressing about one less meal. It makes life a bit simpler and everyone would no doubt like that.

2. Longer Lives.

It is no longer news especially to researchers that one sure way to live longer is through calorie intake restriction. Ordinarily this makes tons of sense. The body has inbuilt within it different interesting mechanisms one of which is the ability to withstand starvation. So when you starve you consciously teach you body to practice the preservation technique. Your body always finds ways to extend your life during starvation. The obvious draw back here is the irony that lies inherent in deliberate starvation for longer lives. We all definitely want a long and enjoyable life but to take the path of starvation in order to achieve this goal is not apparently appealing nor is it appetizing. The bright side of it all is intermittent fasting is able to achieve similar milestones as calorie restriction can since they both can set in motion the process of life extension. So a soft way around this starvation challenge is intermittent fasting. One could even say that this is starvation made simple.

3. Cancer Free.

Fasting has the power to reduce the risk of cardiovascular disease in humans. Full experimentation has not exactly connected the dots tot his claim although individual cases have confirmed the possibility. As regards fasting and cancer, there is still a lot of debate since here too there has not been a lot of research and experimentation done on the relationship between cancer and fasting. The way ahead is not just all bleak because there are glimmers of hope. Early reports hint that the side effects of chemotherapy may be lessened by fasting before treatment. This report is also sustained by another inquiry which arrived at the conclusion that intermittent fasting before any form of chemotherapy results in better cure quotients and invariably fewer deaths. In brief, this wide-ranging revision of various studies on the connection between fasting and disease has arrived at the conclusion that fasting tends to not only take the edge off the risk of cancer, but also cardiovascular disease.

4. Easier Diets.

There are various claims that diets are not effective on the long run so we tend to trust food combination or restriction requirements less but the problem is not inherent in the food selection or restrictions rather it is in the fact that most people hardly ever follow through a diet plan over long terms. Put simply, the problem is not in any way nutritionally based but behavioral in nature. This is where intermittent fasting shines because it's remarkably easy to implement once you get over the idea that you need to eat all the time. For a case in point, one review demonstrated that intermittent fasting was a strategy of use for weight loss in overweight adults and submitted that this is most effective if subjects quickly adapt and remain faithful to an intermittent fasting routine.

5.7 SIDE EFFECTS OF INTERMITTENT FASTING

Intermittent fasting is not suitable for everyone. This is not to discourage anyone but the truth is not all strokes are for every folk. Women who are in the second and third trimesters of pregnancy, for instance, are more at risk and must seek a doctor's advice prior to electing for any form of intermittent fasting. Also people who have medical conditions must seek the counsel of a doctor before they start up any intermittent fasting program. Outside people within these circles, a healthy person would experience very few side effects when they practice intermittent fasting. Physically and mentally sluggishness is a normal reaction while the body attempts to adjust especially at the onset of fasting. After the adjustment, most people go back to functioning normally. More specifically, people at risk from fasting include people who are:

- diabetic

- pregnant

- breastfeeding

- with anorexia

- on medications

- with eating disorders

- attempting to conceive

- with low blood pressure

- Having sugar regulating difficulties

Fatigue

There are persons who want to practice intermittent fasting but because of the rigours of their daily life or exercise regimes they participate in they fear fatigue. Fatigue is a common side effect of intermittent fast and this may lead to loss of muscle mass. The way around this is to step up protein intake during eating periods. For those who indulge in exercise regimes, they must beforehand include specific exercise routine that aim at building resistance. For healthy individuals, intermittent fasting should make them fatigued or affect their ability to exercise only during the period when their bodies are adjusting to the new eating schedule. These ill effects should vanish in subsequent days.

Hunger

It is common to feel your stomach rumble and grumble during your fasting periods especially during the hours close the commencement of the eating period. This experience is more common to people who eat in short intervals. This happens because the body has adapted to the eating patterns. To cut out of this habit, the cycle of stimuli-trigger-reward must be reengineered. Hence the regular cues (stimuli) that are precursors to eating (reward) should be replaced. During fasting periods, it is pertinent to replace looking at, smelling, or even thinking about food, which following normal biological processes initiates the release of gastric acid into your stomach and make you feel hungry or inform the brain that food time is close at hand. In the place of looking, smelling or thinking about food, it is advised that you try reading a book, reducing proximity to food sources or slotting in some mentally absorbing doings.

Binge Eating.

Intermittent fasting from countless reviews is known to always cause a spike in the craving rates of the brain. It has been discovered to remarkably increase cortisol, the stress hormone responsible for cravings. For persons who instinctively resort to eating when stressed the way out of this side effect is to target activities that inhibit the release of the cortisol hormone. These activities could include listening to music, meditating or even yoga. To increase chances of tolerance you must remember to consume nutritious foods and eat to your fill while within the eating period. On no fasting days, if there are in the method chosen, be careful not to binge eat except the intention is to gain weight.

Dehydration.

Intermittent fasting is associated with dehydration because eating goes with drinking and since eating rates or times are cut down, drinking also suffers. It is important to learn to dissociate drinking from eating. Make sure to drink plenty liquids to keep the thirst levels low. Prolonged thirst can lead to the occurrence of other side effects of fasting like fatigue as well. You must keep handy coffee or water or other drinks low in calories during fasting periods.

Tiredness.

This is akin to fatigue although slightly different. When most people fast they try not to engage in any form of activity at all, in fact some prefer to sleep out their fasting periods. This side effect can also strongly cause disarray to usual sleeping patterns. This effect is not forceful for the first timer or within the first week of intermittent fasting. You must be careful not to overlook symptoms such as dizziness and confusion because they suggest that blood sugar levels are low. When symptoms persist, break the fast or see a physician.

PART SIX

6.1   Conclusion

Fasting has been acclaimed to be quite a natural part of the human life. Inadvertently many people have fasted often by having their dinner early and eventually skipping breakfast the next day. Some others have partaken of fasting in a more structured way. On the other hand, it is worthwhile not to neglect the fact that while it is not mandatory that a person remove totally certain food classes from their diet, they must endeavor to eat a balanced diet rich in protein, fiber, and vegetables. Also drink plenty of fluids.

Fasting is widely considered as the conscious abstinence or reduction from all or some of food, drink, or both, for a specified period of time. Fasting can also refer to the metabolic status of a person who has not eaten through the night, or to the metabolic state achieved after full digestion and absorption of a meal. Many people may also fast as a requirement for a medical procedure, such as preceding a colonoscopy or a checkup. Fasting, more broadly, may also be part of a religious ritual. This religious aspect is actually the driving force behind the sustenance of the concept and practice of fasting.

Fasting is mandatorily required prior to surgery, certain medical tests, such as cholesterol testing necessitates fasting for several hours. Fasting often improves mood, alertness, and personal feelings of well-being, perhaps improving overall symptoms of depression. Fasting for durations shorter than 24 hours (intermittent fasting) has been shown to be effectual for weight loss in obese and healthy adults and to preserve lean body mass. Fasting has often been employed as a tool to protest, make a political statement, or to bring awareness to a cause. A hunger strike, a non-violent method of resistance, is often staged as an act of political protest, or to rouse feelings of guilt, or to attain a goal such as a policy change. A spiritual fast presupposes personal spiritual beliefs with the need to express personal principles, from time to time in the context of a social injustice.

There are a couple of myths that are surrounding fasting and these include First is the claim that fasting is simply some new fad or crazy marketing ploy. Fasting has been practiced by people for centuries and its efficacy has repeatedly been affirmed the health benefits of fasting. Second is the claim that fasting is quite foreign to many on the reason that is has never been a trendy topic.

You must realize the most profound of things are hardly trendy topics. Third is the claim that your body is meant to be nourished always. Inadvertently, we all have fasted in one way or another, for one simple reason or out of compulsion; you may just have not realized so. Fourth is the claim that fasting is just perfect and has no side effects. This is quite far from the truth. There are underlying conditions that when we have, fasting would be harmful rather than helpful to us. Final myth claims that when you miss a meal you body is cheated and it will surely bring harm to you. It is true that we need to eat to survive. This does not mean that we live to eat, we only eat to live.

Fasting is a procedure that has been connected with a wide variety of latent health benefits, including weight loss, as well as enhanced brain function, heart health, improved blood sugar control and cancer prevention. There are many different types of fasting that are suitable for nearly every lifestyle, from water fasting to intermittent fasting and calorie restriction. When appended with a nutritious diet and fit lifestyle, integrating fasting into your schedule could greatly benefit your health.

There is an important caveat to be conscious about at all times. Countless research and real life experiences have repeatedly demonstrated and attested to the efficacy of fasting and while it possible to make long list of would-be health reward related to fasting, nevertheless it may not be appropriate for every person. Fasting can pilot occasions of quick rises and unexpected drops in your blood sugar rates, this is particularly true of persons who are plagued by diabetes or low blood sugar, which could be precarious.

Religious fasts as the name suggests are done for spiritual, religious or ritual reasons. The Jewish Tzomot is known to include seven diverse religious fasts through the course of the calendar year. Ramadan is an Islamic fast, lasting one month (this can be consequent 30 days or with breaks but eventually totaling 30 days) during which Muslims fast from break of day to end of the day.

Intermittent fasting is often mistaken to be a form of dieting, it is not a diet; it is a pattern of eating. It is a pattern of eating because fundamentally, it is a way of scheduling the meals you eat in order that you get the largest part out of them. There is the 16/8 method which comprises fasting daily for a minimum of 14 and maximum of 16 hours, and making sure to confine your daily eating period to a minimum of 8 and maximum of 10 hours; the 5:2 diet that requires that special attention is paid to two days out of the seven days of a week; the eat-stop-eat in which there is a full 24 hour fast taken in either of three ways, which is from breakfast to breakfast, lunch to lunch or dinner to dinner; alternate-day fasting denotes fasting every other day. This can be achieved either by not eating anything or restricting eating to only a few hundred calories during the fasting days; the warrior diet that makes provision for a huge meal at dinner time, restrictions come to fore during the day with allowances only for fruits and vegetables; and the form of fasting that is the easiest regime to follow, the spontaneous fast which simply requires that you skip meals from time to time at your pleasure.

Besides weight loss intermittent fast moderates blood pressure, intensifies fat burning and boost neuronal flexibility among other things. Just as fasting, intermittent fasting is not for everyone. Its side effects include fatigue, hunger, binge eating, tiredness and dehydration.

REFERENCES

Norman, Dr (17 April 2003). "Fasting before surgery – Health & Wellbeing". Abc.net.au. Retrieved 18 August 2019.

Russell J &Rovere A, eds. (2009). "Fasting". American Cancer Society Complete Guide to Complementary and Alternative Cancer Therapies (2nd ed.). American Cancer Society. ISBN 9780944235713.

Fond, G; MacGregor, A; Leboyer, M; Michalsen, A (2013). "Fasting in mood disorders: Neurobiology and effectiveness. A review of the literature". Psychiatry Research. **209** (3): 253–8.

Whitney, Eleanor Noss & Rolfes, Sharon Rady (2012). Understanding Nutrition. Cengage Learning. ISBN 978-1133587521.

Shils, Maurice Edward; Shike, Moshe (2006). Modern Nutrition in Health and Disease. Lippincott Williams & Wilkins. ISBN 9780781741330.

Anton, Stephen D; Moehl, Keelin; Donahoo, William T; Marosi, Krisztina; Lee, Stephanie A; Mainous, Arch G; Leeuwenburgh, Christiaan; Mattson, Mark P (2017). "Flipping the Metabolic Switch: Understanding and Applying the Health Benefits of Fasting". Obesity. **26** (2): 254–268.

Leonhardt, David (2013). Nine Habits of

Happiness. DoctorZed Publishing. ISBN 9780980625998.

"Vegetarian Times". Active Interest Media, Inc. 1 October 1985. Retrieved 22 July 2019.

Moore, Jimmy; Fung, Jason (2016). The Complete Guide to Fasting: Heal Your Body Through Intermittent, Alternate-Day, and Extended Fasting. Simon and Schuster. ISBN 9781628600018.

McCue, Marshall D. (2012). Comparative Physiology of Fasting, Starvation, and Food Limitation. Springer Science & Business Media. ISBN 9783642290565.

Espinosa, G. Garcia, M (2008) Mexican American Religions: Spirituality activism and culture. Duke University Press.

Smith, Peter (2000). "fasting". A concise encyclopedia of the Bahá'í Faith. Oxford: Oneworld Publications. ISBN 978-1-85168-184-6.

"The Buddhist Monk's Discipline: Some Points Explained for Laypeople". Accesstoinsight.org. 23 August 2010. Retrieved 18 August 2019.

Randi Fredricks (2012). Fasting: An Exceptional Human Experience. AuthorHouse. ISBN 978-1-4817-2379-4.

Falwell, Jerry (1981). Fasting, what the Bible teaches. Tyndale House. ISBN 9780842308496.

David Grumett & Rachel Muers (2010) Theology on the Menu: Asceticism, Meat and Christian Diet. Routledge.

Gassmann, Günther & Oldenburg, Mark W. (2011). Historical Dictionary of Lutheranism. Scarecrow Press. ISBN 9780810874824.

Ripley, George & Dana, Charles Anderson (1883). The American Cyclopaedia: A Popular Dictionary for General Knowledge. D. Appleton and Company.

Cléir, Síle de (2017). Popular Catholicism in 20th-Century Ireland: Locality, Identity and Culture. Bloomsbury Publishing. ISBN 9781350020603.

Buchanan, Colin (2006). Historical Dictionary of Anglicanism. Scarecrow Press. ISBN 978-0-8108-6506-8.

Kallistos (Ware), Bishop (1964). The Orthodox Church. London: Penguin Books. ISBN 978-0-14-020592-3.

Crowther, Jonathan (2015). A Portraiture of Methodism: The History of the Wesleyan Methodists. T. Blanshard.

Epps, David (2018). "Facts about fasting". The Citizen. Retrieved 16 July 2019.

McKnight, Scot (2010). Fasting: The Ancient Practices. Thomas Nelson. ISBN 9781418576134.

Synan, Vinson (1997). The Holiness-

Pentecostal Tradition: Charismatic Movements in the Twentieth Century. Wm. B. Eerdmans Publishing. ISBN 9780802841032.

Gentilcore, David (2015). Food and Health in Early Modern Europe: Diet, Medicine and Society, 1450-1800. Bloomsbury Publishing. ISBN 9781472528421.

Johnson, William (2003). The Fasting Movement, Bethesda Books.

Griffith, R. Marie. (2000). Apostles of Abstinence: Fasting and Masculinity during the Progressive Era. American Quarterly 52 (4): 599-638.

Nash, Jay R. (1982). Zanies: The World's Greatest Eccentrics. New Century Publishers. ISBN 978-0832901232

Kang, Lydia; Pedersen, Nate. (2017). Quackery: A Brief History of the Worst Ways to Cure Everything. Workman Publishing. ISBN 978-0-7611-8981-7

Fishbein, Morris. (1932). Fads and Quackery in Healing: An Analysis of the Foibles of the Healing Cults. New York: Covici Friede.

ABOUT THE AUTHOR

Doctor Scott is a renowned health experts who has cured many illnesses using natural means.

www.ingramcontent.com/pod-product-compliance
Lightning Source LLC
Chambersburg PA
CBHW070719250726
48662CB00001B/493